Handbook of
Transfusion Medicine

LONDON: HER MAJESTY'S STATIONERY OFFICE

Handbook of Transfusion Medicine

UNITED KINGDOM BLOOD TRANSFUSION SERVICES

Editor:
D B L McClelland

Contributors:
I D Fraser (*Associate Editor*)
J Gillon (*Associate Editor*)
J A J Barbara
F E Boulton
B Brozovic
M Contreras
R J Crawford
H H Gunson
P Hewitt
V J Martlew
W Murphy
J A F Napier
P Trenchard
S J Urbaniak
T B Wallington
P L Yap

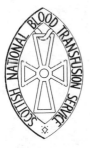

Contents

FIGURES

Preface

This handbook has been produced at the request of the Directors of the UK Transfusion Services, as a successor to the publication "Notes on Transfusion". It is intended for use by medical and other health care personnel, as a source of information about blood component therapy and the clinical use of plasma fractions.

Many colleagues have reviewed the manuscript and provided detailed comments. The help of the following is particularly acknowledged: Dr F Ala, Professor J D Cash, Dr M Contreras, Dr R J Crawford, Dr O B Eden, Dr C Entwistle, Dr R Hume, Dr V Martlew, Dr J F Munro, Dr A J Napier, Dr D Smith, Professor A Spence and Dr W Wagstaff.

Because the field of transfusion therapy is undergoing rapid change, it is intended to update this handbook periodically. We would therefore welcome comments from readers of this first edition.

D B L McClelland
Editor

South East Scotland Regional Transfusion Centre
Royal Infirmary
Edinburgh EH3 9HB

Introduction

Who this book is for

This book is for staff who are responsible for prescribing or administering blood products. It aims to give practical information about the composition and use of these products. A small number of problems account for most of the difficulties and dangers associated with transfusion, for example; delay in obtaining compatible blood when the patient needs it urgently, transfusion of blood which was intended for someone else, over-transfusion leading to heart failure and viral infection from transfused products.

This book is intended to help clinicians to avoid the avoidable risks and to explain those which are unavoidable so they can be taken into account when clinical decisions are made about transfusion for individual patients.

Visiting the blood bank

You should visit the Blood Transfusion laboratory at the start of your hospital appointment. The medical and technical staff will appreciate your interest and will be able to advise and assist you in relation to transfusion therapy for your patients.

The concept of blood component therapy

It is useful for the prescriber to understand a few basic facts about how blood is collected and processed because this affects the safety and availability of the products. *Figure 1* illustrates the processing of blood from donor to patient. Blood is a raw material from which a range of therapeutic products including platelet concentrate, red cell concentrate and fresh plasma are made. Large amounts of plasma are also needed for the production of plasma fractions such as albumin, coagulation factors and immunogloblins. In the United Kingdom most of the plasma is obtained from whole blood donations as shown in the figure. Some is obtained by plasmapheresis.

Blood donors and blood donation testing
Donors can give 450 ml whole blood, generally up to 3 times per year. Donors up to 60 yrs may alternatively give 500-600 ml plasma up to 15 litres per year by plasmapheresis. Platelets and leucocytes can also be collected by cytapheresis.

The medical selection of donors is intended to exclude anyone whose blood might harm the recipient, for example by transmitting infection. In the UK every blood donation is tested for evidence of Hepatitis B, HIV-1 and Syphilis. In other countries, different tests for infection may also be needed, depending on the frequency of infections in the community. Each donation is tested to determine the blood group (ABO and Rh D group).

Preparation of blood components
Blood is collected into sterile plastic packs which can be centrifuged to permit separation of red cells, platelets and plasma in a closed system. These are called **blood components**. They are stored in and supplied from the blood bank (*Figure 1*). Plasma prepared in this way or obtained by plasmapheresis may be further processed into plasma fractions.

Manufacture of plasma fractions
Plasma fractions are partially purified therapeutic preparations of plasma proteins. They are manufactured, usually in a large scale pharmaceutical process, from large

volumes of pooled donor plasma. Typically the plasma from up to 20,000 individual donations will be mixed to give about 5000 kg of bulk plasma (*Figure 2*). Processing involves mixing with ethanol and varying temperature, pH and ionic strength conditions to precipitate different groups of proteins. Further purification steps are carried out and fractions are then freeze dried or stored in solution.

Plasma from any one of the large number of individual donors who contribute to each batch of product could potentially introduce infectious organisms into the process so careful screening of every donation is vital. Even with screening, some viruses may find their way into the pooled plasma, so it is important that the process includes stages to inactivate any infectious agents which might escape detection. More detail is given in the descriptions of individual products.

Cost of products
Although blood is donated freely in the UK, the processing to specialised products is expensive. Plasma fractions are also available from commercial sources. The cost of these products is shown in *Table 9* and should be borne in mind when making treatment decisions.

Implications of the consumer protection act (1988)
On March 1st 1988, the new consumer protection act became law. This legislation changes and extends the basis on which a patient might make a successful legal claim following infection or some other adverse reaction associated with a transfusion. It may be some time before the full implications of this act for transfusion practice are worked out. It is important for staff who prescribe and

administer blood products to ensure that they are familiar with the product descriptions and safety data contained in this handbook and that local practices for prescribing and administration take adequate account of this information. **Where package inserts are provided these should be read and acted upon as for any other drug.**

Labelling
All blood products must be clearly labelled and users should understand the significance of the label information. The label should state the details of the product and its composition, the conditions under which it can safely be stored and the date and time of expiry. Blood components from single donors must carry the unique donation number which identifies that donation. (This can be used to check back to the complete record of that individual donor.) Plasma fractions must carry a unique batch number which should allow the manufacturer to trace all the original donations in that batch.

Blood components issued to individual patients will normally also carry a compatibility label, giving the details of the patient for whom the component is intended (*Page 30*).

Immunological compatibility
All blood components containing red cells must be labelled to show their ABO and Rhesus D (Rh D) group. It is not routine to test for other red cell antigens. All red cell containing components must be compatible with the ABO and Rh D group of the recipient. The compatibility requirements for other blood products are given in Section 2.

Procedures for ordering and administering blood components

Because of the need for compatibility testing it is essential to adhere to thoroughly documented procedures to ensure that there is no risk that any patient can receive an incompatible blood component.

If you do not know the relevant procedures for your hospital, you are most strongly advised to read the procedure manuals and to make sure that you understand them before you order blood components or set up a blood component infusion on any patient.

Most serious accidents arising from blood component administration are caused by failure to comply with standard procedures in the ward or theatre environment.

General procedures for ordering and administering blood are given in *Section 3*. This should be read by any staff required to carry out these tasks.

Blood components and plasma fractions

Terminology

In this book the term **blood products** is used for all therapeutic materials made from blood and includes both blood components and plasma fractions. The term **blood components** refers to red cell preparations, platelet concentrate, fresh plasma and cryoprecipitate. These are usually issued in packs containing the components prepared from a single blood donation or pooled together from a small number of donations.

The terms that are used for each of the blood components and the information given about them have been specified by a joint working party of the National Institute of Biological Standards and Control and the Blood Transfusion Services. These specifications and terms will be adopted for blood components throughout the UK. However there will be a transitional period during which some blood components will continue to be labelled with slightly different terms. Where relevant, these are given with the product descriptions.

Plasma fractions are the plasma protein preparations produced from bulk pooled donor plasma.

As with any other medicines, sensible prescribing and use of blood products is based on knowledge of their composition, properties and side effects. This section gives this information and it is referred to throughout the later sections of this book.

Red cell components

Whole blood

CPD-Adenine-1 Whole Blood (Human).

Unit of issue: 1 donation, also referred to as a ''unit'' or ''pack''.

Description: Approximately 510 ml volume (450 ml donor blood and 63 ml anticoagulant). Haematocrit 35-45%. No functional platelets or granulocytes.

Infection risk: Not sterilised, so capable of transmitting any agent present in cells or plasma which has not been detected by routine donor screening, including Hepatitis B, Hepatitis Non A Non B, HIV-1 and other viruses.

Storage: Between 2C and 6C in an approved blood refrigerator fitted with a temperature chart and alarm.

May be stored up to five weeks if collected in a suitable anticoagulant such as citrate phosphate dextrose with added adenine (CPDA1). During storage, changes in composition occur resulting from red cell metabolism. These include a fall in pH, rise in plasma potassium and fall in red cell content of 2, 3 Diphosphoglycerate (2, 3 DPG) which impairs the release of oxygen to tissues for a few hours after the red cells are infused. Although most clotting factors are relatively stable in storage, Factors V and VIII fall to 10-20% of normal during the first two weeks.

Administration: Must be ABO and Rh D compatible with the recipient.

Indications: Whole blood should not be used routinely for red cell replacement.

Its **use should be restricted** to situations where replacement of plasma proteins as well as red cells is needed.

Precautions: Whole blood should not be given to patients

with chronic anaemia who have a normal or elevated plasma volume.

Fresh whole blood: (Usually defined as blood less than 24 h after collection.) There are insufficient scientific data to define clinical indications for its use. Blood that has not undergone full microbiological testing should not be considered safe for transfusion.

Red cell concentrate

Plasma Reduced Blood, Concentrated Red Cells.

Unit of issue: 1 donation.

Description: About 200 ml red cells from which most of the plasma has been removed to give a PCV of 55-75% (usually about 65%).

Infection risk: Same as whole blood.

Storage: Same as whole blood.

Administration: Same compatibility requirement as whole blood. To improve flow, sodium chloride IV infusion 0.9% BP (50-100 ml) may be added using a Y-pattern giving set.

Indications: Replacement of red cells in anaemic patients. Used with saline or colloid solution to replace acute blood loss.

Red cell concentrate, supplemented

Red Blood Cells, Optimal Additive System.

Unit of issue: 1 donation.

Description: About 200 ml red cells with minimal residual plasma to which saline adenine glucose solution or equivalent red cell nutrient solution has been added. Haematocrit 50-70%. Better flow rate than red cell concentrate.

Infection risk: As whole blood.

Administration: As whole blood.

Indications: As red cell concentrate.

Precautions: In UK not currently advised for neonates or for exchange transfusion. If patient is at risk of volume overload the additive solution can be removed following centrifugation before administration.

Red cell packs for paediatric use
Transfusion centres may supply packs containing small volumes (usually 100 ml) of red cell preparations for children.

Leucocyte depleted red cell components

There are several different methods of preparing leucocyte-depleted blood or red cells. Most transfusion centres supply these products, or they may be prepared in the hospital blood bank.

Infection risk: As whole blood but probably reduced transmission of CMV. The risk of bacterial contamination limits approved storage period to 24 h after processing.

Indications: Patients who have leucocyte antibodies and who have experienced two or more previous febrile transfusion reactions.

Minimise HLA immunisation in patients receiving repeated transfusion.

May reduce risk of CMV transmission in special situations (*see Pages 57, 69*).

Red cell concentrate, leucocyte depleted, filtered
Leucocyte Poor Blood, Filtered.

Red cells from which most of the plasma has been removed and more than 95% leucocytes have been removed by filtration.

Leucocyte removal by filtration at time of infusion
Filters are available which can be used in the infusion line

during administration. These filters will remove 95% or more of leucocytes from stored units of whole blood or red cell concentrate.

Red cell concentrate, washed

Leucocyte Poor Blood, Saline Washed.

Red cells from which most of the plasma, leucocytes and platelets have been removed by washing. At least 97% of plasma protein should be removed.

Red cell concentrate (thawed and washed)

Red Blood Cells, Thawed and Washed.

Unit of issue: 1 donation.

Description: Red cells can be preserved by freezing in liquid nitrogen vapour using a cryopreservative. Recovery of these frozen cells is a specialised procedure. Up to 20% of the red cells are lost during recovery. The product supplied for use contains negligible amounts of leucocyte fragments and plasma proteins. After infusion, the red cells should have a similar survival in the circulation to conventionally stored red cells.

Storage: In the frozen state 10 years. After thawing and washing maximum 24 hours at 2C-6C.

Infection risk: As leucocyte poor red cells.

Indications: Uses should be strictly limited due to high cost. Storage of autologous units for patients in whom compatible blood would be very difficult to obtain.

Storage of red cells of rare groups for potential patient use.

Platelet components

Platelet concentrate

Unit of issue: May be supplied either as a single donor unit or as a pack containing a pool (usually of 4 to 6 donor units).

Description: Single donor unit; volume 50-60 ml of plasma containing at least 55×10^9 platelets with some red cells (usually $< 1.2 \times 10^9$/unit) and leucocytes ($< 0.12 \times 10^9$/unit).

Infection risk: As for whole blood but **a normal adult dose involves 4 to 6 donor exposures.**

Storage: 20C to 24C (with agitation) for 5 days (some centres use packs which restrict storage to 72 hours). **After pooling,** platelets must be infused within 4 hours. Must not be refrigerated.

Administration: 4 to 6 platelet units (which may be supplied pooled) should be infused through a standard blood administration set over a period of less than 30 mins. Use a fresh giving set, primed with saline. Do not give through a set which has already been used for blood. Platelets prepared from Rh D positive donors should not normally be given to Rh D negative potential child-bearing females. Ideally platelets of the patient's own ABO group should be given. If platelets of a different ABO group are used the contained plasma may cause a positive direct antiglobulin test (but rarely haemolysis) in the recipient.

Indications: Bleeding due to thrombocytopenia or platelet functional defects.

Prevention of bleeding in thrombocytopenia due to marrow failure.

Treatment of microvascular bleeding in patients transfused with large volumes of blood (*Page 51*).

NOT indicated for prophylaxis of bleeding in surgical patients unless known to have significant pre-operative platelet deficiency.

Dose: In a 60 or 70 kg adult, 5 or 6 single donor units

should raise the platelet count by 20-40 $\times$ 10^9/l (increment will be less if there is splenomegaly, DIC or septicaemia).

Complications: Reactions (fever or urticaria) are not uncommon, especially in multi-transfused patients. For management see Section 1.

Platelet concentrate (cytapheresis)
Unit of issue: 1 pack containing platelets collected by cytapheresis from a single donor.

Description: Volume 150-300 ml. Platelet content 150-500 $\times$ 10^9, equivalent to 3-10 single donations. **Note that platelet content, volume of plasma and leucocyte contamination vary widely depending on the collection procedure.**

Infection risk: As whole blood.

Storage: Up to 24 hours at 20-24C (with agitation) unless collected using a system validated for longer storage periods.

Administration: As for random donor platelets.

Indications: For patients with HLA antibodies who are refractory to random platelets. Platelets from a single HLA compatible donor are indicated.

Non HLA matched cytapheresis platelets can be used for the same indications as random donor platelets.

Leucocyte depleted platelet components

Platelet concentrate, pooled and filtered
A pool of random donor platelets which have been filtered to remove at least 95% of leucocytes.

Partial leucocyte removal ($>$85%) may also be achieved by centrifugation using specially designed packs.

Leucocyte removal by filtration at the time of infusion
Filters are available which can be used in the infusion line.
These will remove > 95% of leucocytes with moderate loss
of platelets.

Indications: Patients with leucocyte antibodies who
experience severe febrile transfusion reactions.

Minimise HLA immunisation in patients receiving
repeated platelet transfusion.

May reduce CMV transmission in special situations (*see
Pages 57, 69*).

Leucocyte components

Leucocytes (cytapheresis)
Unit of issue: Usually a single donor apheresis collection.
Description: Volume 200-300 ml (mainly plasma). Should
contain at least 10×10^9 granulocytes and will have a
variable content of red cells, lymphocytes and a substantial
platelet content. Depending on method of collection may
also contain Dextran or hydroxyethyl starch.

Leucocyte concentrate may also be prepared from whole
blood donations by separation of the "buffy coat" fraction
which contains leucocytes together with large amounts of
platelets and red cells. Each unit will contain 0.5 to 1.5 $\times$
10^9 leucocytes.

Infection risk: As whole blood.

Storage: Without agitation, at 20-24C. Should be used as
soon as possible after collection and not later than 24
hours.

Administration: Because of high red cell content, red cell
compatibility testing is necessary. HLA compatibility is not
generally required. Since granulocyte recipients are often
immunosuppressed it is usual to irradiate the product
before administration (1500-2500 cGy) to avoid Graft v

Host disease. Potential bone marrow recipients should not receive granulocytes from the proposed bone marrow donor. Transfuse over 2-4 hours using a standard blood giving set, with careful clinical monitoring to detect reactions which are frequent. Hydrocortisone (100 mg IV) and Chlorpheniramine (10 mg IV) may be given prior to infusion to reduce the severity of reactions. Daily infusions over at least four days are usually advised.

Indications: Controversial and changing. Use of granulocyte infusions is declining due to evidence that early and aggressive antibiotic treatment may be more effective. Collection of granulocytes has a significant risk of complications for the donor and is expensive.

Use should only be considered if the patient has:

Absolute granulocyte count $< 0.5 \times 10^9/l$.

Fever or proven infection which is not responding to appropriate antibiotic therapy including anti-fungal agents given for at least 48 hours.

A reasonable chance of survival for some time if supported through the acute episode.

Complications: Severe reactions are not infrequent. Up to 15% of recipients have fever. Severe lung reactions may occur in patients with active lung infections.

Plasma components

Fresh frozen plasma

Unit of issue: Pack containing plasma separated from one donation and frozen within 6 hours of collection. Packs containing smaller volumes may be available for children.

Description: Volume 200-250 ml. Contains normal plasma levels of stable clotting factors, albumin and immuno-globulin. Factor VIII level at least 70% of normal fresh plasma level (ie 0.7 iu/ml or more).

Infection risk: As whole blood but low risk of transmitting cell associated virus eg HTLV-1.

Storage: At −30C or below for up to 1 year. After thawing infuse as soon as possible. If delay is unavoidable, hold at 2-6C. If used as a source of labile coagulation factors, must be infused within 6 hours of thawing.

Administration: Must normally be ABO compatible to avoid lysis of recipient red cells but no compatibility testing (crossmatching) is needed. After thawing at 37C in the blood bank, infuse as soon as possible using a standard blood giving set. Clinical monitoring is essential as reactions are not uncommon. Occasional severe life threatening anaphylactic reactions occur.

Indications: Replacement of multiple clotting factor deficiencies in patients with liver disease or who are overdosed with coumarin anticoagulants (*Page 61*).

In patients receiving large volume transfusions who develop microvascular bleeding (*Page 51*). For these indications, an initial dose of 12-15 ml/kg (4 packs for a 60 kg adult) is appropriate.

Thrombotic thrombocytopenic purpura.

Pseudocholinesterase deficiency.

C1 inhibitor deficiency.

Precautions: **Fresh frozen plasma should not be used as a volume expander or as a source of nutrition. Much safer products exist for these requirements.**

Fresh frozen plasma (paediatric unit)
The fresh frozen plasma in a pack containing 50 ml, for use in children.

Fresh frozen plasma (apheresis)
Unit of issue: Single apheresis donation containing approximately 500-600 ml.

Other plasma preparations: (These may be available from some centres.)

Plasma (cryoprecipitate depleted): Plasma from which approximately half the fibrinogen, FVIII and fibronectin has been removed as cryoprecipitate but containing the other plasma constituents.

Single donor plasma: Plasma separated soon after collection but not rapidly frozen or plasma separated at any time up to five days after expiry of whole blood unit.

Cryoprecipitate

Unit of issue: For adults usually supplied as a pool of 6 or more single donor units in one pack.

Description: Prepared from fresh frozen plasma by collecting the precipitate formed during controlled thawing, and resuspending it in 10-20 ml plasma. Contains about half of the Factor VIII, fibrinogen and fibronectin in the donation. Eg Fibrinogen 150-300 mg/pack, FVIII 80-100 iu/pack.

Infection risk: As for plasma but a normal adult dose involves at least 6 donor exposures.

Storage: At −30C or below for up to 1 year. After thawing infuse as soon as possible. Must be infused within 6 hours of thawing.

Administration: Use ABO compatible product if possible but no compatibility testing is needed. Pooling needs to be done carefully to avoid loss, since the volume in each pack is small. Wash packs out with a small volume of sodium chloride 0.9%. Infuse through a standard blood administration set. If possible complete infusion within 30 mins.

Indications: As an alternative to Factor VIII concentrate in the treatment of inherited deficiencies of von Willebrand Factor (von Willebrand disease), FVIII and Factor XIII.

Replacement of fibrinogen in patients who are bleeding due to low fibrinogen (< 0.5 g/l).

Treatment of DIC.

Has been used as a source of fibronectin in management of severe bacterial infections but the value of this therapy remains unproved.

May be useful in bleeding in uraemic patients.

Plasma fractions

Factor VIII concentrate

Unit of issue: Vials of freeze dried protein labelled with content, usually about 250 iu.

Description: Partially purified factor VIII prepared from large pools of donor plasma. Factor VIII ranges from 0.5-20 iu/mg of protein. These products are all heated or chemically treated to inactivate HIV-1.

Infection risk: Current virus inactivated products do not transmit HIV-1. Hepatitis risk of current heat treated products is reduced substantially.

Storage: Unless otherwise indicated on the manufacturer's package insert, freeze dried powder should be kept at 2-8C up to stated expiry date. Once the powder is dissolved the solution should be drawn up using a filter needle and must be infused within 2 hours.

Administration: The product is reconstituted according to manufacturer's instructions and infused either through a standard giving set or butterfly needle.

Indications: Treatment of Haemophilia A.

Treatment of von Willebrand's disease.

Factor IX concentrate (prothrombin concentrate)

Unit of issue: Vials of freeze dried protein labelled with content, usually about 350-600 iu of Factor IX.

Description: Partially purified Factors II, IX and X. Some preparations contain Factor VII also. Prepared from large pools of donor plasma. Heated or chemically treated to inactivate HIV. Hepatitis viruses may also be inactivated.

Infection risk: As Factor VIII.

Administration: As Factor VIII.

Indications. Treatment of Haemophilia B (Christmas Disease).

Immediate correction (if required) of very prolonged prothrombin times in Coumarin overdose if patient cannot tolerate required volume of Fresh Frozen Plasma.

Treatment of Haemophilia A with inhibitors.

Contra-indications: Not usually advised in liver disease as some Factor IX products may have a risk of thrombosis and DIC. Transmission of Hepatitis viruses is especially hazardous to these patients.

Coagulation Factor concentrate for treatment of patients with inhibitors to Factor VIII. Two commercially manufactured licensed products, *Feiba* and *Autoplex* are available in the UK.

Description: A heat treated plasma fraction containing partly activated coagulation factors which support haemostatic activity in patients with inhibitors to Factor VIII. The nature of the coagulant activity is not yet fully characterised.

Infection risk: Probably the same as other heat treated factor concentrates.

Storage: As factor VIII concentrate.

Administration: As Factor VIII concentrate.

Indications: Patients with inhibitors to Factor VIII. **Should be used only with specialist advice.**

Immunoglobulin preparations

Normal human immunoglobulin

Description: Made by cold ethanol fractionation of large

pools of human donor plasma. It contains antibody to measles, mumps, varicella, hepatitis A and other viruses and bacteria currently prevalent in the donor population. Protein concentration 150 g/l of which at least 95% is IgG. Traces of IgA and IgM are present. Vials of 5 ml containing approximately 750 mg IgG or of 1.7 ml containing 250 mg.

Specific human immunoglobulins

Description: Made by cold ethanol fractionation from plasma donations selected to contain high levels of specific IgG antibodies (obtained from convalescent patients or from donors recently immunised with the relevant vaccine). Protein concentration 100-150 g/l. Vial content varies according to product.

Infection risk: Intramuscular Immunoglobulin preparations correctly manufactured by standard cold ethanol fractionation have an excellent safety record and transmission of HIV and Hepatitis NANB has not been reported with this type of product.

Storage: 2-6C within the labelled shelf life.

Administration: By deep intramuscular injection.

Side effects: Are very unusual (other than pain at injection site).

Indications: Intramuscular preparations of normal or specific immunoglobulin are used for prevention of infections (*Page 73, Table 8*).

Treatment of antibody deficiency states.

Precautions: **Do not give intravenously.** Do not give to patients with IgA deficiency who have antibody to IgA.

Rh D immunoglobulin

Unit of issue: Dose units of 250 iu or 500 iu. Larger vials (2,500 iu or 5,000 iu) may also be available. **N.B.** The antibody content of anti Rh D products may be stated in iu or ug: 5 iu is equivalent to 1 ug.

Description: Prepared from plasma containing high levels of anti Rh D antibody. Products made in the UK are for intramuscular administration. Intravenous preparations are manufactured commercially.

Indications: Rh D immunoglobulin prevents the development of antibodies to Rh D positive red cells introduced into the circulation of an Rh D negative individual. Its principal use is in the prevention of haemolytic disease of the newborn (*Page 59*).

Human immunoglobulin for intravenous administration
Description: A liquid or freeze-dried preparation made from pools of human donor plasma by cold ethanol fractionation and subsequent processing to render product safe for IV administration. Vial content usually 3 g, 6 g or 12 g. Protein concentration after reconstitution 30-50 g/l. Licensed preparations contain a stabiliser eg sucrose (2 g/g of IgG).

Infection risk: Cases of Non A Non B hepatitis have occurred in recipients of IV IgG preparations which are not currently licensed in the UK. Biochemical evidence of hepatitis has also been reported in recipients of licensed products. There is no evidence of transmission of HIV.

Storage: 2-6C according to manufacturer's labelled shelf life, although some lyophyllised preparations can be stored up to 25C.

Administration: IV infusion according to manufacturer's product insert. **Initial infusion rate should be slow** since reactions are more common with first infusion and with fast infusion rates, especially in hypogammaglobulinaemic patients.

Side effects: In 5-10% of infusions, headache, nausea, tachycardia, hypotension, malaise, angioedema, urticaria and fainting may occur. Usually alleviated by slowing or stopping infusion. Prior administration of antihistamine or aspirin may avoid. There have been isolated reports of severe systemic infection, coagulation disturbances and haemolysis of red cells following high dose IV IgG.

Indications: Idiopathic thrombocytopenic purpura.

Other immune cytopenias.

Hypogammaglobulinaemia.

Other Immunological disorders.

Human albumin solutions

Unit of issue: See *Table 1.*

Description: Albumin is prepared by fractionation of large pools of blood donor plasma. Albumin is typically supplied as 4.5% or 20% solutions, in a variety of dose units. A product similar to 4.5% Albumin is available from some manufacturers as Stable Plasma Protein Solution (SPPS) or Plasma Protein Fraction (PPF).

Infection risk: No risk of transmitting viral infections.

Administration: No compatibility requirements. No filter needed.

Indications: 4.5% Albumin (and SPPS, PPF). Acute blood volume replacement (*Page 49*).

Burns: after the first 24 hours (during which saline may be advised) 4.5% albumin may be used to maintain plasma albumin near 25 g/l and a colloid osmotic pressure above 20 mm Hg.

As exchange fluid in therapeutic plasmapheresis.

In patients in which severe acute albumin losses are sustained eg small bowel infarction and acute pancreatitis.

Albumin 20%. These preparations are hyperoncotic and expand the plasma volume at the expense of the extra vascular compartment. They may be useful in:

short term management of hypoproteinaemic patients

(eg with liver disease) who are fluid overloaded and resistant to diuretics.

diuretic resistant patients with nephrotic syndrome. In these situations, 20% Albumin should be used with a diuretic.

Precautions: Administration of 20% Albumin may cause acute expansion of intravascular volume with risk of pulmonary oedema. Any albumin solutions are more likely to precipitate pulmonary oedema than are crystalloids. **Do not use for IV nutrition. A very expensive and inefficient source of essential aminoacids.**

Table 1 Albumin Solutions

Product	Composition				Examples of dose units
	Albumin content	Protein g/l	Sodium mmol/l	Potassium mmol/l	
SPPS or PPF	83% of Total Protein	40-50	<160	<2	400 ml: 16-20g protein: up to 64 mmol Na
Human Albumin 4.5%	96% of Total Protein	40-50	<160	<2	500 ml: 20-25g protein: up to 80 mmol Na 100 ml: 4-5g protein: up to 16 mmol Na
Human Albumin 20%	96% of Total Protein	150-250	<160	<10	100 ml: 15-25g protein: up to 15 mmol Na 5 ml: approx. 1g protein: <1 mmol Na

Note that precise formulations and dose units may differ between manufacturers of these products.

Non plasma colloid volume expanders

Albumin solutions are currently widely used as first line acute volume expanders. This practice is not justified as much less expensive synthetic products are readily available and equally effective. Once these synthetic products have been used in the recommended doses (see below) and further sustained volume expansion is required then the introduction of an albumin solution may be justified.

Solutions of large molecules such as Dextran, or modified gelatin provide an inexpensive source of fluid with a colloid osmotic pressure similar to that of plasma. These molecules remain in the plasma for shorter periods than albumin and lack its transport functions. Acute allergic or anaphylactoid reactions have been reported but are very rare. *Table 2* lists some important features of these products.

Synthetic colloid solutions are frequently used as part of standard initial resuscitation regimes. The low incidence of life threatening anaphylactic reactions (of the order of 5-10/100,000 infusions) combined with the lack of infection risk and low cost argue in their favour. Dextrans produce a haemostatic defect, in part by impairing platelet function. Provided doses are kept within 1.0-1.5 g/kg body weight (equivalent to 1 to 1.5 litres of Dextran 70 for an adult) bleeding time is not adversely affected. **Dextran can make blood grouping and compatibility testing difficult so samples for this purpose should be taken before the infusion is started.**

Table 2 Non Plasma Colloid Volume Expanders

Product	Source	Concentration of solution	Number average Mol. wt.	Intravascular persistence	Approximate frequency of severe acute reactions
Modified gelatin	Heat-degraded cattle bone gelatine	3-4%	35,000	50% of infused volume persists 4-5 hours	1 in 10,000 infusions
Hydroxy-ethyl starch (HES)	Maize starch, chemically modified	6%	450,000 or 265,000	Similiar to or longer than Dextran 70	1 in 20,000 infusions
Dextran 70	Bacterial product	6%	70,000	50% of infused volume persists 24 hours	1 in 10,000 infusions
Dextran 40	Bacterial product	10%	40,000	Shorter than Dextran 70	1 in 50,000 infusions

Procedures

Ordering and administering blood

Most transfusion deaths are due to clerical mistakes when samples are taken from the patient or when blood is administered. The practical precautions given in this section are therefore extremely important.

If you do not know the procedures for your hospital, you are most strongly advised to read the relevant procedure manuals and to make sure that you understand them before you order blood components or set up a blood component infusion on any patient.

Samples and request forms for compatibility testing

i. **Identify the patient accurately.** Read the wrist band and whenever possible ask the patient to state his/her forename, family name, and date of birth. Check this information against the casenotes or pre-printed patient identification label. **Follow the local procedure manual. Unconscious patients MUST be identified by the information given on the identity band.**

ii. **Emergency casualties who cannot be reliably identified must be given an identity band with a unique number. This number must be used to identify this patient until full and correct personal details are available.**

iii. Fill in the patient's details clearly and accurately on the blood request form. Label the **sample tube** at the patient's bedside, clearly and accurately.

iv. State on the request form the quantity of blood which is required.

v. State the time the blood is needed. Avoid requesting blood "as soon as possible". This does *not* help the blood bank staff to determine priorities. Comply with local rules about the timing of blood orders for planned procedures.

vi. **Take full personal responsibility for ensuring that the blood sample from the patient is placed in the correct tube for that patient. Your signature on the request form and tube label implies that you have ensured that the sample is accurately identified.**

vii. Send an adequate blood sample to the laboratory (for adults, usually 10 ml, no anticoagulant) in the type of specimen tube used locally for transfusion samples.

Blood ordering in an emergency

Procedures for identification of the patient and labelling of tubes and forms must be strictly followed.

The blood bank should be informed as quickly as possible of the quantity of blood needed and the time it is needed. Special transport arrangements may be required.

In some situations the blood bank may advise the use of Group O blood, but usual practice in the UK is to provide blood of the patient's ABO and Rh D group. This can usually be issued within 15 minutes of the blood bank receiving a patient's blood sample. Local arrangements vary. If your job is likely to involve urgent blood ordering you must make yourself familiar with the local system.

Blood ordering for planned procedures

Blood banks usually offer two stages of readiness to meet expected blood needs. These are:—

1. *Group and screen.* (Sometimes called *group and hold*). The

patient's ABO and Rh D group is determined and serum is tested for the presence of unexpected red cell antibodies. The patient's serum sample is then normally stored in the laboratory for up to 7 days (check local variations). If blood is urgently needed it can be provided safely for the patient after a rapid procedure to exclude ABO incompatibility. Using this method the blood bank will need 10-15 minutes to have blood ready for issue to the patient.

This procedure avoids the need to set aside blood units for a given patient and so allows better use to be made of a limited blood bank stock.

2. *Crossmatch (compatibility test)*. In this procedure the patient's ABO and Rh D group is determined. In addition, the patient's serum is screened for the presence of any unexpected antibodies to red cells. The patient's serum is then tested directly for compatibility with the red cells of the units of blood to be transfused. Compatible units of blood are then labelled specifically for the patient and may be issued or held in the blood bank for immediate issue on request.

If further blood is required for a patient who has been recently transfused, a fresh sample must be sent for crossmatching.

Crossmatching problems *Priorities when a patient has a red cell antibody:* The blood bank must receive an adequate sample (usually 10 ml clotted blood for an adult) in an accurately labelled tube. The patient's red cells must be tested to determine the ABO and Rh D group. The patient's serum should be screened against carefully selected standard red cells using sensitive methods to identify any red cell antibodies of potential clinical importance. (In practice these are, IgG antibodies which are active at 37C). If such antibodies are found, testing against a larger panel of standard red cells will be needed to identify the antibody, and specially selected red cells will be required.

When a clinically significant red cell antibody is found in a patient's serum, every effort will be made by the transfusion laboratory to provide blood which is negative for the corresponding antigen, to avoid the risk of a haemolytic reaction or of boosting the antibody to a high level. However, this may involve a lot of laboratory work and considerable delay.

When a patient needs transfusion urgently and it is anticipated that there will be delays in finding compatible blood, the physician responsible for the blood bank should be asked to advise on the likelihood of a severe or fatal adverse reaction if incompatible blood is given. **This risk must be balanced with the risk of delaying transfusion when a patient's life is at serious risk from blood loss.**

Blood order schedule
Blood requirements for surgical procedures can be predicted from analysis of previous use. Many surgical procedures virtually never need transfusion and there is no need to involve the blood bank. Examples are tonsil and adenoid removal, varicose vein stripping and hernia repair.

The *group and screen* procedure should be used for surgical procedures where blood is rarely required. For procedures that predictably require blood replacement it is usual to order a pre-determined number of crossmatched units to be available for surgery. This request should equal the number of blood units that meet the transfusion needs of 90% of similar procedures (based on an analysis of previous operations).

Each surgical unit should have a **blood order schedule or tariff** based on actual blood use. This should be used as the basis for blood ordering.

Release, collection and storage of blood

Depending on the local system, blood may be released by the transfusion laboratory on request or it may require to be collected directly from a designated blood refrigerator by authorised staff.

The person collecting the blood must bring documentation which specifies the patient's identification details. At the time of collection a check must be made that these details match those of the blood unit to be collected. There should be a written record of the issue or collection of each pack.

Blood must be kept refrigerated. If a pack is withdrawn from refrigeration and if infusion is not commenced within 30 minutes, it is no longer suitable for further clinical use. In this event the pack should be labelled according to the local procedure and returned to the transfusion laboratory.

Administering blood

Check identities

Local procedure manuals must specify the identification checks to be carried out and designate the staff who may perform and sign for them.

Blood supplied from the blood bank should have a compatibility label firmly attached. This should carry the following information:

Family name of patient.
First name or initial.
Date of birth or hospital number.

Patient's group.
Unique number of pack.
Time for which blood is requested.

At the time of transfusion the information on the compatibility label attached to the blood product must be checked carefully with the patient's identification, including the patient's wrist band.

No discrepancies in spelling of the patient's name or in the patient's identification number should normally be accepted.

Observe the patient

The patient should be carefully observed for the first 5-10 minutes after the infusion starts. If possible give the first 50 mls of each unit slowly since the first part of each blood unit infused serves as an *in vivo* compatibility test. The patient's condition including pulse and temperature must then be checked and recorded periodically according to the local procedure manual until the transfusion is complete. Clinical features of acute transfusion reactions are given in *Section 4*.

Record keeping

Details of all blood components infused (including the donation numbers) must be entered into the patient's case record together with the compatibility report provided by the transfusion laboratory.

Time limits for infusion

There is a risk of bacterial proliferation if blood or red cell packs are kept at room temperature. For this reason the infusion must be started within 30 minutes of removing the pack from refrigeration and should normally be completed within 4 hours of removing the pack from

refrigeration. The giving set should be changed at least 12 hourly during blood infusion. For other products, guidance is given in the product descriptions.

Blood administration sets
All blood components must be infused through a set containing an integral filter (170 um) to trap large aggregates.

Microaggregate filters
Filters of 20-40 um pore size can trap small aggregates of leucocytes and platelets which form in all blood stored beyond 5-10 days. There is no indication for using these filters with small volume (2-4 units) transfusions in an adult. Even with very large transfusion volumes there is no proof that microaggregates cause respiratory problems. These filters should be used in patients transfused during cardio-pulmonary bypass and may be useful in large volume transfusion of patients with pre-existing lung disease. For exchange transfusion of neonates blood less than five days old should be used, thus microaggregate removal should not be necessary.

Blood warmers
There is no evidence that warming blood is beneficial to the patient when infusion is slow (1-3 units over several hours). At infusion rates greater than 100 ml/minute cold blood may cause cardiac arrest. Blood warmers must have a visible thermometer and an audible warning device. Red cells and plasma are altered at temperatures over 40C and can cause severe transfusion reactions. **Blood must NOT be warmed by putting the pack into hot water or on a radiator or near any uncontrolled heat source.**

Use of blood warmers should be limited to adults receiving

infusion of large blood volumes at rates greater than 50 ml/kg/hr, children receiving volumes greater than 15 ml/kg/hour and exchange transfusions in infants.

Simultaneous administration of other drugs and fluids
Red cell concentrate may be diluted with sodium chloride 0.9% to improve the flow rate. This is most simply done if a Y pattern giving set is used. **No other solutions should be added to any blood component.** They may contain additives such as calcium (Ringer's lactate). This can cause citrated blood to clot. Dextrose solution (5%) can lyse red cells.

Drugs should never be added to blood components; if there is an adverse reaction it will be impossible to determine if this is due to the blood, to the medication which has been added or to an adverse interaction of the two.

Autologous transfusion

Since immunological and infective complications can result from donor blood, the alternative of using the patient's own blood may be considered in suitable cases. This approach may also be of value in situations of blood shortage.

Immediate pre-operative bleeding and haemodilution: This procedure is often used in cardiothoracic surgery. Immediately before operation, blood is withdrawn with appropriate fluid replacement and stored, refrigerated, in the theatre. During or after surgery, the patient's blood can be reinfused. This procedure allows the patient's haematocrit to be reduced to a level selected for optimal capillary perfusion.

Intra-operative blood salvage: During surgery with significant bleeding into the operative field, the patient's blood may be collected by suction. The blood is then washed to produce a suspension of the patient's red cells suitable for re-infusion. This method may be particularly useful for cardiothoracic procedures. Trained staff and specialised equipment are required.

Pre-operative bleeding with liquid storage of the patient's blood. Patients who are awaiting planned surgery may donate blood to be stored for use during or after their operation. Their blood can be stored for up to 5 weeks using standard blood bank conditions. **Medical selection must ensure that patients are fit for this procedure.** Suitable patients can lay down 2-4 units of blood pre-operatively. Before retransfusion, autologous blood units must be grouped for ABO and Rh D and be crossmatched to avoid the consequences of any possible clerical errors. Pre-deposit blood should not be transfused to anyone other than the patient who provided the donation. Detailed guidelines for this procedure are available (*see Further Reading*).

Long-term frozen storage of autologous donations: Frozen red cells can be stored for long periods. This permits autologous red cell donations to be stored for a planned procedure. Frozen blood storage is expensive and the facilities are available only in a few regional transfusion centres.

There are some practical limitations to the application of auto-transfusion. Not all patients are fit enough to have 450 ml of blood withdrawn several times before a planned operation. Auto-transfusion does not reduce the risk of errors that can cause ABO incompatible transfusion. Therefore autologous transfusion requires the same careful procedures used in requesting, labelling, testing and administering donor blood.

FOUR

Adverse effects of transfusion

As with all forms of therapy the risk of transfusion must be weighed up against the benefit which each individual patient will obtain, when deciding to prescribe blood or blood products. This section indicates the frequency and severity of the major adverse effects of transfusion, how to avoid them or how to manage these problems when they occur. An overview is given in *Table 3*.

Acute transfusion reactions

It is important to monitor the patient closely for at least the first 5-10 minutes of the infusion of each unit of blood to detect early clinical evidence of acute reactions.

Acute intravascular haemolysis (eg ABO incompatibility) See Table 5 on page 43 for summary of investigation and management.

The main features of acute haemolytic reactions are shown in *Table 4*. Major haemolytic reactions are very rare but potentially lethal. Pyrexial and urticarial reactions may occur in at least 2% of transfusion recipients.

A major haemolytic reaction is almost always due to the infusion of ABO incompatible blood. The reaction is usually most severe if Group A blood is infused to a Group O patient. These reactions are almost always due to clerical errors (either the wrong blood is put into the crossmatching tube, or there is a failure to carry out the basic check of the blood pack with the patient's identity band).

Table 3 Acute and Delayed Complications of Transfusion

Problem	Cause	Timing in relation to transfusion	Frequency of occurrence	Severity of resulting clinical condition; management
ACUTE COMPLICATIONS				
Acute intravascular haemolysis of transfused red cells.	ABO mismatched transfusion. Group A into Group O is worst.	Often during first few ml of infusion.	Very rare. 1 death per 34,000 patients transfused (Honig & Bove 1980).	Mortality high due to DIC and acute renal failure. *Treat:* see Table 5. *Prevent:* use safe documentation and checking systems for blood administration.
Anaphylactic reaction to plasma-containing products	Antibodies to IgA Other—not characterised.	During infusion.	Extremely rare: IgA deficiency with IgA antibody occurs in <1 in 10,000 population.	Mortality high as for other severe anaphylactic reactions. *Treat:* acute anaphylaxis. *Prevent:* don't transfuse any IgA containing product to these patients.
Fever/Rigors	Anti-leucocyte antibodies in patient who has been pregnant or transfused.	Towards end of infusion or within hours of completing infusion.	0.5-1% of transfusions (but usually in previously transfused patients).	Unpleasant. *Treat:* Aspirin. *Prevent:* use a leucocyte depleted red cell product.

Table 3—Continued Acute and Delayed Complications of Transfusion

Problem	Cause	Timing in relation to transfusion	Frequency of occurrence	Severity of resulting clinical condition; management
Urticaria	Patient antibodies to infused plasma proteins.	During infusion.	1-2% of transfusions.	Unpleasant. *Treat*: temporarily stop infusion and give Chlorpheniramine 10-20mg. *Prevent*: pre-medicate with Chlorpheniramine 10-20mg before transfusion.
	Infusion of allergens which react with patient IgE antibody.			
Pulmonary Oedema Congestive cardiac failure	Excessive rate of volume of infusion.	During infusion.	Not known.	Dependant on clinical situation; prevention and treatment as standard clinical practice.
Non Cardiogenic pulmonary oedema.	Donor plasma containing antibody to patient's leucocytes: aggregates trapped in lungs.	During or shortly after infusion.	Rare: ? a special problem in therapeutic plasmapheresis with FFP replacement.	Life threatening. *Treat*: respiratory support, diuretics and high dose steroids. *Prevent*: transfuse with leucocyte depleted washed red cells.
	Recipient plasma antibodies to transfused leucocytes.			

Table 3—Continued Acute and Delayed Complications of Transfusion

Problem	Cause	Timing in relation to transfusion	Frequency of occurrence	Severity of resulting clinical condition; management
Infective Shock	Red cells, whole blood or platelets contaminated with bacteria. Commonly Pseudomonas fluorescens; Staphylococcus may contaminate platelets.	Usually during infusion of first 100 mls of contaminated pack.	Very rare— Approx. 1 report per year.	Very high mortality *Treat:* manage septicaemia. Gentamicin 3-5 mg/kg 8 hourly PLUS Cepalothin 1-2g 4 hourly or other appropriate antibiotics.
DELAYED COMPLICATIONS				
Delayed haemolysis of transfused red cells.	Red cell allo-antibodies eg JK^a, Fy^a, K.	3-10 days after transfusion.	Not known	Reduces survival of transfused red cells.
Post transfusion purpura.	Most cases due to antibody to PlA1 in patient who is PlA1 negative.	2-14 days after transfusion.	Very rare (PlA1 negative = 2.4% population)	May be life threatening. *Treat:* high dose IV IgG usually with steroids.

Table 3—Continued Acute and Delayed Complications of Transfusion

Problem	Cause	Timing in relation to transfusion	Frequency of occurrence	Severity of resulting clinical condition; management
Allo-immunisation	Transfusion of red cells which are not of same phenotype as the patient. White cell and platelet antibodies usually after repeated transfusion.	Days to weeks after infusion.	Variable: anti Rh D will develop in at least 75% of Rh negative patients given Rh positive blood.	Avoid transfusion of Rh D positive cells to Rh D negative recipients.
			1-5% of previously transfused patients have red cell antibodies. More than 10% repeatedly transfused patients have white cell and/or platelet antibodies.	Leucocyte depleted red cells and platelets may reduce incidence.
Increased risk of tumour recurrence (?)	Not known	Evident as a late effect.	Not known. All data from retrospective studies.	No prospective study to demonstrate effect on mortality or morbidity.

Table 3—Continued Acute and Delayed Complications of Transfusion

Problem	Cause	Timing in relation to transfusion	Frequency of occurrence	Severity of resulting clinical condition; management
Iron overload	One unit of red cells contains 250mg of iron. Accumulation is very likely over a long course of transfusion.	Clinical manifestations after some years of regular transfusion.	Usual in transfusion dependant patients.	Severe morbidity due to haemosiderosis. *Prevent* or delay by chelation therapy.
Viral infection transmitted by blood products	See page 46.			

Table 4 Early Clinical Features of Intravascular Haemolytic Transfusion Reactions

Dyspnoea	Fever
Chest pain	Chills
Flushing	Back pain

Oliguria
Hypotension
Generalised oozing and
  bleeding from puncture
  sites and surgical wounds.

Haemoglobinaemia
Haemoglobinuria

Many of these features may be inapparent in an anaesthetised patient. With ABO incompatible blood, signs and symptoms may appear after 5-10 ml of the infusion. Prognosis is much worse if 200 ml or more has been given.

The incompatible red cells lead to the activation of the complement and coagulation systems. Shock, disseminated intravascular coagulation and renal damage are likely to result. It can be very difficult at the bedside or in the operating theatre to decide if the patient is having a life-threatening intravascular haemolytic reaction. *Table 4* lists the features which may suggest severe haemolytic reaction but many of these may be absent in an unconscious or anaesthetised patient. In practice, **if an ABO incompatible transfusion is suspected, the transfusion must be stopped and urgent steps taken to confirm or exclude this possibility** (*see Table 5*).

Haemolytic reactions due to other antibodies

Antibodies such as Rh (D, C, c̄, E, ē) Kidd (Jkᵃ), Duffy (Fyᵃ) and Kell lead to destruction of transfused red cells which takes place mainly in the spleen or liver. A moderate fever, falling haemoglobin and rising bilirubin

Table 5 Management of Suspected Haemolytic Transfusion Reaction

Investigation	*Therapy*
1. **Double check the labelling of the blood unit with the patient's ID band and with other identifiers.**	1. **Stop blood. Keep IV open with sodium chloride 0.9%.**

2. Take 40 ml of blood for labs.
  — Blood bank   5 ml anticoagulated
                    5 ml clotted
  — Clin Chem   10 ml electrolytes
  — Coag Lab   10 ml coag screen
  — Bacteriology   blood culture
	2. **Catheterise bladder and monitor urine flow.**
	
	3. **Give Frusemide 150 mg IV.**

Blood bank should be asked to report immediately the plasma haemoglobin and direct antiglobulin test result.	4. **Give saline 100-200 ml. Give Mannitol (20%) 100 ml if no diuresis occurs after frusemide.**
Compatibility testing will be repeated using pre and post transfusion serum samples.	5. **Insert CVP line and give sodium chloride 0.9% to maintain CVP between +5 and +10 cm water.**
The blood pack(s) will be examined to exclude bacterial contamination as a cause of the transfusion reaction.	6. If urine flow 2 hours after Mannitol and Frusemide is <100 ml/h assume acute renal failure and obtain specialist help. 7. If urine flow >100 ml/h adjust infusion rate to maintain this.
3. ECG — ? evidence of hyperkalaemia.	8. If hyperkalaemic, check electrolytes (? metabolic acidosis). If venous bicarbonate <20 mmol/l give isotonic sodium bicarbonate 100-200 ml, then give 50 ml glucose with 8 units of insulin (rapid IV) followed by 10% dextrose with 12 units of insulin over 4 hours. Rectal resonium A may be needed also.
4. Arrange repeat coagulation screens and biochemistry 2-4 hourly.	9. If DIC give blood product support (platelets and cryoprecipitate). 10. If patient needs transfusion use rematched blood. There is no increased risk of a second haemolytic reaction.

will be accompanied by a positive direct antiglobulin test in the patient. Haemolysis may be severe, leading to renal failure. This type of reaction may occur quickly, or may be delayed up to 10 days following transfusion until red cell antibody production is stimulated leading to destruction of the transfused red cells. In the latter case the term **delayed haemolytic transfusion reaction** is used. These delayed reactions may pass unnoticed.

Febrile reaction

Fever or rigors during transfusion may suggest acute intravascular haemolysis but more frequently is due to antibodies against white cells. The transfusion should be stopped and the blood unit (and patient sample) sent to the transfusion laboratory for investigation. Symptoms usually respond to aspirin (0.6-0.9 g). Recurrent severe febrile transfusion reactions may be prevented by the use of leucocyte poor blood.

Allergic reactions

Most allergic reactions consist of urticaria and itch occurring within minutes of starting the transfusion and settle with an antihistamine (eg chlorpheniramine 10-20 mg, by intramuscular or slow intravenous injection). The transfusion may be continued if there is no progression of symptoms after 30 minutes.

Chlorpheniramine (10 mg parenterally) may be given before transfusion when a patient has previously experienced repeated allergic reactions.

Very rarely, life-threatening reactions occur which may be associated with antibodies against IgA. They may be prevented by the transfusion of washed red cells or products collected from donors who are IgA deficient.

Severe Anaphylaxis

Requires urgent resuscitation—full details are given in the British National Formulary.

First line treatments for anaphylactic reactions include

- maintain airway and give oxygen,
- give chlorpheniramine 10-20 mg by slow IV injection over at least 1 minute,
- administer salbutamol by nebuliser,
- if there is no improvement, further therapy must be given according to the patient's condition. Expert help must be sought.

Hypervolaemia Fluid overload occurs when too much blood is transfused or the transfusion is too rapid. Acute left ventricular failure occurs with dyspnoea, hypertension and tachycardia, This requires standard medical treatment including intravenous diuretic therapy and administration of oxygen. The transfusion should be stopped or slowed. Volume overload is a special risk with 20% Albumin solutions.

Patients with chronic anaemia are normovolaemic or hypervolaemic and may already have signs of congestive cardiac failure. This may require diuretic therapy accompanying blood transfusion. Red cell concentrate should be used. Each unit should be given slowly over 2-4 hours at a time when the patient can be closely observed. Normally not more than one unit should be given in each 12 hour period

Iron overload

Transfusion dependant patients receiving red cells over a long period become overloaded with iron. Chelation therapy (with Desferrioxamine) is used to minimise accumulation of iron.

Infectious agents transmitted by transfusion

The risk that a blood component or plasma fraction can transmit an infectious agent depends on its prevalence in the community, the effectiveness of the processes used to exclude and detect infected donors and the processes used to sterilise the product. **For a patient receiving a non sterilised blood component, the risk will depend on the number of individual donors to whom the recipient is exposed.**

Hepatitis B

Donations are screened for Hepatitis B surface antigen (HBsAg). Despite this, Hepatitis B is occasionally transmitted by transfusion because the donor may be in the early phase of infection before antigenaemia has become detectable by screening tests. Reports of Hepatitis B infection in recipients suggest a frequency of 0.2% or less. Evidence of Hepatitis B infection is common in patients who have regularly received coagulation factor concentrates.

Hepatitis Non A Non B

No serological screening test is yet available to detect the responsible viruses, although this may be introduced in the foreseeable future. Tests on donors for Hepatitis B core antibody and elevated liver enzymes are used in some countries and may provide some reduction in post transfusion hepatitis.

The true incidence of post transfusion hepatitis is very difficult to establish because many cases are not reported and most cases are asymptomatic and detectable only by prospective studies which monitor liver enzyme levels. **Clinical** NANB hepatitis is reported in the UK with a frequency of about 1 in 30,000 units of blood transfused. Studies to detect **asymptomatic** hepatitis on blood component recipients suggest a frequency of 1-2.5% in the UK, the Netherlands and Sweden. Much higher rates have been reported from the USA. Most patients who have received non-heat treated coagulation factor concentrates have evidence of infection with Non A Non B Hepatitis.

HIV-1

All blood donations are screened for antibodies to HIV-1. The prevalence of infection among donors in the UK is about 1 in 70,000 (in the USA about 1 in 10,000). A very small proportion of infective donors may fail to be detected because antibody has not yet developed at the time of testing. The risk of infection being transmitted by a tested blood component has been estimated at around 1 in 300,000 units transfused in the UK and is probably substantially less than this.

HTLV-I

This virus causes neurological disorders and adult T-cell leukaemia. It is transmissable by the transfusion of cellular blood components. Prevalence is high in some parts of Japan and the Caribbean. Prevalence in blood donors in the United Kingdom is not yet known. The risk of transfusion transmitted disease is not yet known but is probably very small.

CMV

Prevalence of antibody is approximately 50% in UK donors. It is not known what proportion of these can transmit the virus through transfusion. Transfusion transmitted CMV is probably clinically important in premature infants weighing less than 1200 g who are born to CMV sero-negative mothers; also in CMV sero-negative bone marrow graft recipients who receive CMV sero-negative grafts. For these patients CMV sero-negative blood components should be given.

Treponemal infections

All donations are screened for serological evidence of treponemal infections. The infectivity of Treponema pallidum declines as blood is stored at 2-6C. Risk of transfusion transmission in the UK is extremely small.

Malaria

In the UK donor selection is designed to exclude potentially infectious donors from donating red cells for transfusion and reports of transfusion transmitted malaria are extremely infrequent. In endemic areas the administration of antimalarial drugs to blood recipients may be necessary.

Clinical applications of blood products

This section deals with some clinical situations in which the use of blood and blood products may be an important part of management. Many of these situations involve complex conditions which should be managed by clinicians with specialist training and experience.

Massive blood loss

Replacement of acute blood loss
This section refers to situations where urgent administration of blood is necessary for the patient's survival. The objectives are:—

i. **intensive early treatment to restore circulating volume and avoid hypoperfusion.** This is the key to avoiding late severe complications of shock;

ii. **control of bleeding and maintenance of adequate blood oxygen transporting capacity.**

Treat haemorrhagic hypotension promptly: (*Table 6*) Insert a large IV cannula, collect blood for grouping and infuse saline or a mixture of saline and a colloid volume expander as rapidly as possible until an acceptable blood pressure is reached. After about 40% of the estimated blood volume has been infused (30-35 ml/kg), 4.5% albumin can be introduced to comprise 50% of the total infusion volume. This offers the benefit of maintaining plasma colloid osmotic pressure. However, the clinical benefits of this product (rather than saline) have not been clearly established. Red cell concentrate or whole blood should be infused as soon as available.

Hypovolaemia with low blood pressure and poor tissue perfusion is the patient's greatest enemy. The priority is to give *any* intravenous fluid quickly, and enough to maintain normal circulation. The restoration of haemoglobin level and the maintenance of colloid osmotic pressure are normally of secondary importance.

Table 6 Replacement of acute blood loss

Blood loss		Preferred replacement material
% Vol*	Vol (l)	
<20%	1	Sodium chloride 0.9%
20-40%	1-2	Sodium chloride 0.9% or non plasma colloid + red cells
40-90%	2-5	Whole blood, or red cells with Sodium chloride 0.9% or 4.5% Albumin
>90%	>5	Whole blood. (If bleeding continues and laboratory tests of haemostasis are abnormal, platelets, plasma or cryoprecipitate may be needed)

* Blood volume 70 ml/kg, eg 5000 ml for adult of 70 kg (10 units of whole blood)

Note that 5% albumin solution cost 50-100 times more than saline solutions. Clinical trials in humans have not demonstrated that albumin solutions are superior to saline for resuscitation.

Ordering blood in an emergency: Procedures for identification of the patient and labelling of tubes and forms must be strictly followed.

The blood bank should be informed as quickly as possible of the quantity of blood needed and the time it is needed. Special transport arrangements may be required.

In some situations the blood bank may advise the use of Group O blood, but usual practice in the UK is to provide ABO and Rh (D) compatible blood. This can usually be issued within 15 minutes of the blood bank receiving a transfusion sample.

Haemostasis in recipients of large volume transfusions
Haemostatic problems may be partly due to dilution during blood loss and replacement but the main causes are tissue damage, hypoxia, and sepsis. These lead to consumption of platelets and coagulation factors. Some patients, such as neonates, those with marrow disorders, or liver disease and those on anticoagulant therapy have reduced reserves of platelets or clotting factor production and are more likely to develop haemostatic problems.

Blood component replacement: When there is no underlying medical complication, replacement of up to one blood volume (8-10 units of blood in an adult) with red cells and non-plasma fluids is not likely to be associated with haemostatic problems. To replace larger volumes stored whole blood provides adequate replacement of fibrinogen and other stable clotting factors. The reduced level of Factor V and Factor VIII in these donations does not lead to functional clotting deficiencies in the recipient. As an alternative to stored whole blood, red cell concentrate together with fresh frozen plasma may be used but this exposes the patient to a greater number of donors, increasing the risk of virus transmission.

Laboratory tests of coagulation: These help to identify patients who need blood components to control microvascular bleeding.[1] A platelet count $< 50 \times 10^9$/l, fibrinogen < 0.5 g/l or prothrombin time ratio (INR) or

Footnote
Definition of microvascular bleeding (MVB). Bleeding from mucous membrane; oozing from catheter sites which persists after application of pressure; continuous oozing from surgical wound and raw tissue surfaces; generalised petechiae or increased size of ecchymoses.

APPT ratio greater than 1.8 are strongly associated with microvascular bleeding. These tests should be monitored during large transfusions and used to guide replacement when bleeding occurs.

Platelet replacement: Is indicated when there is microvascular bleeding (especially if more than 15 units of blood have been replaced) or if there is additional laboratory evidence of disseminated intravascular coagulation.

Fibrinogen replacement: In DIC, fibrinogen replacement may be required in addition to giving platelets. Fresh frozen plasma contains about 0.5 g per donor unit. Cryoprecipitate contains about 0.15-0.3 g of fibrinogen in 15-20 ml as well as other factors which may be important in correcting the haemostatic defect. For an adult, transfusion of 16 packs of cryoprecipitate (containing 3-4 g fibrinogen) should raise the fibrinogen level by at least 1 g/l. Repeated administration may be needed and will be judged both on laboratory data and clinical course.

Cryoprecipitate or plasma infusions should be given when microvascular bleeding is associated with a fibrinogen below 0.5 g/l. Coagulation tests may be prolonged due to a fibrinogen level below 0.5 g/l but a prolonged PT or APPT when the fibrinogen is above 0.8 g/l suggests a deficiency of Factor V and VIII requiring the administration of fresh frozen plasma.

There is no clear evidence that giving platelets or plasma prophylactically to patients undergoing large transfusions reduces the risk of MVB. Routine prophylactic use of these products is therefore not recommended.

Expert advice: The blood replacement management of these patients is often complex and requires substantial resources. You should seek advice from the physician in the Blood Bank or Haematology Service.

Respiratory and metabolic complications of large volume transfusions

Since these problems are unlikely to be due only to transfusion, they cannot be avoided simply by attention to transfusion practice but care should be taken not to make the problems worse.

Adult respiratory distress syndrome: The risk is minimised if good perfusion is maintained while over-transfusion is avoided. The use of albumin solutions to maintain a plasma oncotic pressure greater than 20 mm Hg is often stated to be important but controlled studies on the resuscitation of patients have not established an advantage of albumin solution over crystalloid fluids. The use of microaggregate filters when stored blood is transfused is often advised but the benefits remain unproven. These filters may offer benefit for patients with pre-existing lung disease.

Hypocalcaemia: Citrate in anticoagulants binds ionised calcium and could lower plasma levels, but rapid liver metabolism of citrate normally avoids this. In **neonates** and **hypothermic** patients hypocalcaemia together with hyperkalaemia may be cardiotoxic. If there is ECG or clinical evidence of hypocalcaemia, a dose of 5 ml of 10% calcium gluconate (for an adult) should be given IV and repeated if necessary till the ECG is normal.

Hyperkalaemia: The plasma in a unit of stored whole blood may contain 5-10 mmol of potassium. Combined with hypocalcaemia, acidosis and hypothermia this additional potassium can lead to cardiac arrest. These problems are best prevented by **avoiding hypothermia.**

Acid base disturbances: Despite the lactic acid content of transfused blood, adequate resuscitation involving transfusion usually improves acidosis in a shocked patient and transfused citrate can contribute to metabolic alkalosis in large volume transfusions.

Hypothermia: Rapid transfusion of blood at 4C can lower the core temperature by several degrees. Hypothermia in conjunction with the other metabolic changes mentioned may lead to cardiac arrest. A blood warmer should be used in adults receiving large volumes of blood at infusion rates above 50 ml/kg/hr (in children, above 15 ml/kg/hr).

Perioperative transfusion—the trigger for red cell replacement

Surgical and anaesthetic practice has tended to be guided by the belief that a haemoglobin level below 10 g/dl (haematocrit below 30%) indicates a need for perioperative red cell transfusion. There is little or no firm evidence supporting this belief and experience in recent years suggests that patients with severe anaemia may tolerate anaesthesia and operation without major morbidity or mortality resulting from anaemia itself. Evidence from clinical and physiological studies does not support the necessity for the ''10 g/30% rule''. Experimental evidence indicates that in healthy humans cardiac output does not increase dramatically until the haemoglobin falls below 7 g. Healthy anaesthetised primates survive a haematocrit down to 5% when breathing oxygen.

The decision to transfuse red cells to an individual patient should take account of the duration of anaemia, the

procedure to be carried out, the extent of likely blood loss, and the presence of co-existing conditions such as myocardial ischaemia, pulmonary disease, and cerebral vascular disease.

As a guide, patients who are otherwise healthy with a haemoglobin of 10 g/dl or greater, rarely require perioperative transfusion. Acute anaemia with a haemoglobin below 7 g will generally require red cell transfusion. Some patients with chronic anaemia, such as those with chronic renal failure, tolerate haemoglobin values below 7 g and withstand anaesthesia and surgery at this level. The decision to transfuse red cells will depend on clinical assessment and may require laboratory data such as arterial oxygenation, oxygen extraction ratio and blood volume.

Transfusion for anaemia in the absence of active bleeding

Chronic anaemia

The cause of anaemia must be diagnosed and treatment with haematinics given where appropriate.

Patients who have become chronically anaemic have a deficit of red cells but not of blood volume. In such patients, volume overload is an important hazard.

If red cell replacement is clinically indicated, red cell concentrate should be used. A rapid rise in haemoglobin is not normally necessary in such patients. Rapid infusion increases the risk of volume overload. Elderly patients with chronic anaemia, particularly those with cardio-respiratory disease, should not normally receive more than one unit of red cell concentrate each 12 hours. A diuretic such as frusemide should be given with the transfusion if there is thought to be a risk of circulatory overload.

Transfusion dependent conditions

Patients with transfusion dependent conditions such as myelodysplastic syndromes, haemoglobinopathies and aplastic anaemia may require regular transfusion of red cells over a long period. These patients require specialist management and their transfusion regimes must be designed to minimise problems such as iron overload, and the development of antibodies to red cells and leucocytes.

Transfusion of the newborn

The newborn infant has a small blood volume (80 ml/kg ie 200 ml in a 2.5 kg infant) and the bone marrow responds more slowly than the adult. Repeated bleeding for diagnostic tests can readily lead to anaemia. Some neonates are at special risk of infection. These factors must influence transfusion practice.

Products available: Some centres provide small volume packs of red cells (50-150 ml) and fresh frozen plasma (50-100 ml). Others supply standard donation units. In this case, the required volume of product should be given over a maximum of 4 hours and the remainder returned to the blood bank. **Partly used packs must be returned to the blood bank or discarded to avoid the risk of re-use.**

Some neonatal units still use "walking donors" (often staff members) who donate 10-50 ml of blood to be given directly to an infant. This practice should be discouraged. Donor testing, record keeping and quality control are likely to be inadequate. An adverse reaction to a transfusion of this type could lead to problems related to product liability.

It is usual to supply blood or red cells less than seven days old for neonates to provide maximum oxygen transport capacity, a minimum burden of potassium and freedom from microaggregates. However in most circumstances, blood stored for somewhat longer periods will be safe and effective.

Compatibility testing: The normal rules of ABO and Rh compatibility apply. However since infants under 4 months rarely make antibody to red cells it is not necessary to crossmatch repeatedly if several transfusions are needed. For infants up to 4 months, maternal blood can be used for crossmatching provided the ABO groups are compatible since IgG antibody in the infant's circulation will be derived from the mother. Some centres provide Group O Rh negative routinely for neonates of mothers known to have no atypical red cell antibodies while others supply ABO and Rh matched blood. It is important to be familiar with the local practice.

Platelets: A single donor platelet concentrate should normally produce an acceptable platelet increment in children under 10 kg bodyweight. If the plasma volume (up to 70 ml per platelet concentrate) is excessive, the blood bank should be asked to remove plasma to a minimum volume of 10-15 ml per platelet concentrate.

CMV infection: Premature infants whose mothers do not have antibody to CMV may be infected with CMV if transfused with a unit that is CMV sero-positive. For these infants it is desirable to transfuse blood, red cells, platelets or plasma obtained from donors who are known to be CMV sero-negative at the time of donation. Infants who are not immunosuppressed do not require to be given CMV negative components.

Irradiated blood components: Some centres advise that blood components which contain lymphocytes should be irradiated to avoid a theoretical risk of graft **versus** host disease in premature infants. Present evidence does not support routine use of irradiated products for neonates.

Alloimmune neonatal thrombocytopenia: This is usually due to maternal antibodies to the platelet antigen Pl^{A1}. There may be a history of thrombocytopenia in previous infants. Thrombocytopenia may be severe and require platelet replacement. Platelets may be obtained from the mother and washed to remove plasma containing the antibody or from compatible platelet donors when the specificity of the antibody is known. Mother's platelets are best collected by plateletpheresis using a cell separator. High dose intravenous IgG therapy may be an alternative treatment (*Page 72*).

Thrombocytopenia with maternal ITP: Maternal IgG antiplatelet antibodies cross the placenta so platelet transfusion of the infant is of limited value. High dose IV IgG therapy can be used to raise the infant's platelet count. Administration of high dose IV IgG to the mother before delivery may also be effective (*Page 72*).

Exchange transfusion: Blood for exchange transfusion should be compatible with the mother's serum and should be ABO group compatible with the infant. The blood should be crossmatched against the mother's serum. Red cells less than 7 days old with a haematocrit of 50-60% should be used. Red cells suspended in nutrient solution such as SAG Mannitol which are deficient in plasma are not currently advised for exchange transfusion.

Intrauterine transfusions: A fetus severely affected with haemolytic disease of the newborn (HDN) may require intra-uterine transfusion. This may be given by infusion into the peritoneal cavity or under ultrasound or fetoscopic control by direct transfusion into the umbilical cord. Red cells given should be less than 7 days old, Group O Rh negative and compatible with the mother's serum, a CMV antibody negative donation should be selected if possible. The PCV should be 70% or more to minimise the volume load. Irradiation of the red cells is usually advised to avoid the risk of graft **versus** host disease.

Haemolytic disease of the newborn (HDN)—prevention

Mechanism of HDN: Haemolytic disease of the newborn is caused by destruction of fetal red cells by maternal IgG antibodies directed against red cell antigens which are inherited from the father. The mother may develop antibodies due to fetomaternal haemorrhage during pregnancy or during delivery or as a result of previous transfusion. HDN varies in severity from death in utero to mild anaemia.

Antibody to the Rh D antigen is the most important cause of HDN but is now uncommon in the UK due to the effectiveness of prophylaxis with Rh D immunoglobulin. Although ABO incompatibility between mother and fetus is common, clinically significant HDN rarely results. Other blood group antigens which can elicit IgG antibodies (Kell, Duffy, Rh c) are infrequent causes of HDN. IgM antibodies do not cause HDN because they do not cross the placenta.

Antenatal screening: Pregnant women should be screened to identify Rh D negative mothers, and those who already have antibodies which could cause HDN.

A blood sample taken at the antenatal booking visit should be ABO and Rh grouped and screened for unexpected antibodies. When IgG antibodies are found a sample of blood from the father should also be obtained for red cell typing as this may help predict the risk of HDN.

If no antibodies are found, Rh D negative mothers should have a repeat antibody screen at 28-30 weeks of gestation.

If anti D is found in the first sample regular samples should be obtained throughout the rest of the pregnancy to monitor antibody levels.

Use of Rh D immunoglobulin:

i. **Rh D immunoglobulin must be given postnatally to an Rh D negative mother if her infant is Rh D positive.**

The standard dose is 500 iu. This is sufficient for a fetomaternal haemorrhage of 4-5 ml of red cells.

A Kleihauer test should be done to determine the number of fetal red cells in the mother's circulation. For bleeds larger than 5 ml of red cells, extra anti Rh D IgG must be given (100-125 iu for each 1.0 ml of red cells).

Rh D immunoglobulin by IM injection should be given within 72 hours of delivery but even if a longer period has elapsed it may still give protection and should be administered.

ii. **Rh D immunoglobulin should be given in other situations where an Rh D negative mother may be exposed to fetal red cells.**

Fetomaternal haemorrhage may occur with stillbirths, abortions (including therapeutic abortion) or threatened abortions, amniocentesis, chorionic villus sampling, external cephalic version and after abdominal trauma (eg seat belt injury) or antepartum haemorrhage.

Rh D negative mothers should routinely be given anti D following these incidents. Up to 20 weeks gestation 250 iu should be given at the time of the incident. From 20 weeks on 500 iu should be given.

iii. Rh D immunoglobulin can also be used to prevent immunisation if for any reason blood components containing Rh positive red cells have to be given to an Rh D negative woman under 45 years of age. The dose is calculated to clear the estimated quantity of red cells given. **Despite the availability of effective prophylaxis, up to 20% of Rh D negative women who still develop anti D do so simply because of failure to administer Rh D immunoglobulin postnatally or after an abortion. Efficient administration of the HDN prevention programme is essential to avoid this serious clinical problem.**

Haemostasis and transfusion

Normal haemostasis depends on four systems: soluble pro-coagulant proteins (the coagulation cascade), the platelets, the fibrinolytic system, and the blood vessel wall. **Acquired haemostatic disorders** arise frequently in hospital practice. Blood component therapy is often essential and the choice and dosage of blood component must be based on correct interpretation of clinical features and laboratory tests.

Management of **congenital coagulation defects** such as haemophilia A and B and von Willebrand's disease needs the close co-operation of a specialist.

Acquired haemostatic disorders
Acquired coagulation defects that often contribute to bleeding in hospital practice are dealt with in this section.

Footnote
The antibody content of anti D products may be stated in micrograms (ug) or in international units (iu).

$$1 \text{ ug} = 5 \text{ iu}$$

Liver disease: The haemostatic abnormalities may be complex and include reduced synthesis of pro-coagulant proteins and fibrinolytic inhibitors. Other problems may include activation of coagulation and fibrinolytic systems and platelet deficiency due both to under production and to sequestration in an enlarged spleen. Replacement of blood components can provide only transient improvement in haemostasis.

In massive bleeding in patients with liver disease blood components play a part in supportive therapy. Whole blood should be used to replace blood loss. Platelet transfusions should be given perioperatively. Coagulation factor deficiencies should be replaced with fresh frozen plasma. Factor IX concentrates are currently not generally recommended because of the risks of hepatitis in patients with existing liver disease, but newer heat treated concentrates may carry a lower risk than multiple doses of plasma. Frequent monitoring of platelet count, prothrombin time ratio (INR) and fibrinogen may be necessary as it is not possible to predict the doses of products required.

In patients with a prolonged prothrombin time it is usual to attempt correction of the prothrombin time ratio to 1.5 or less prior to **liver biopsy** or other elective procedures by giving vitamin K parenterally and infusing using fresh frozen plasma; platelet concentrates may also be given to thrombocytopenic patients but in the presence of hypersplenism they are unlikely to be of value.

Uraemia: The bleeding tendency results from an impaired interaction between platelets and the vessel wall to form the primary haemostatic plug. Platelet transfusions have limited benefit but bleeding may be controlled or prevented by red cell transfusion to raise the haematocrit above 30%, or by infusion of cryoprecipitate. Administration of DDAVP or oestrogen may also help in the prevention and treatment of uraemic bleeding, possibly acting by improving the interaction of platelets with the vessel wall. The routine laboratory test which helps in managing these patients is the bleeding time which should be corrected to normal before elective procedures such as renal biopsy are undertaken.

Disseminated Intravascular Coagulation: The essential lesion is the generation of active thrombin in the circulation leading to consumption of circulating pro-coagulant factors. Often there is intravascular fibrin deposition that results in organ damage.

The treatment in every case is to remove the cause where possible and to reverse the deficiencies of clotting factors and platelets. Where the volume infused is not critical, fresh frozen plasma and platelets should be given. Where hypofibrinogenaemia is profound, cryoprecipitate should be infused (an initial adult dose of 10-12 packs) to raise the fibrinogen above 1.0 g/l. In situations where there is a danger of fluid overload, prothrombin concentrate (Factor II, IX and X or Factor II, VIII, IX, X) should be given with platelets and cryoprecipitate.

Antithrombin III concentrates may prove to be an important therapeutic option in DIC. Heparin therapy is rarely indicated.

The diagnosis of DIC is established by detecting the presence of fibrin (ogen) degradation products in the presence of prolongation of the thrombin time, prothrombin time ratio (INR) and partial thromboplastin time. Hypofibrinogenaemia may be present; thrombo-cytopenia is usual. The coagulation screen should be used to monitor clotting factor consumption and the effects of replacement.

Coumarin (Warfarin) overdose: Coumarin anticoagulants (eg Warfarin) interfere with synthesis of Factors II, VII, IX and X. Over-anticoagulation should be managed according to the prothrombin time ratio (INR) and whether there is active bleeding or a need to reverse anticoagulation prior to urgent surgery or an invasive procedure.

INR > 2 with haemorrhage. Give Vitamin Kl, 2.5-10 mg by slow intravenous injection with infusion of fresh frozen plasma or of Factor II, IX and X concentrate. Some Factor IX preparations do not contain Factor VII: the addition of FFP may be needed to correct the INR if these are used.

INR 4.5 to 7 but no haemorrhage. Withhold Warfarin.

INR > 7 but no haemorrhage. Withhold Warfarin. Vitamin Kl, 5-10 mg by mouth (adult dose) may be needed.

An adult may require 2-4 packs of FFP or more to produce any significant shortening of the INR. If there is a risk of circulatory overload, Factor II, IX, X concentrate would be indicated, in an initial dose of 1-2 vials (600-1200 units of Factor IX) with monitoring of the INR. Vitamin K1 may take up to 12 hours to act: larger doses tend to act more rapidly. After a large dose of Vitamin K1, it can be difficult to re-establish anticoagulation with oral agents.

Thrombolytic therapy—management of excessive bleeding. Streptokinase, urokinase and plasminogen activator cause fibrinolysis by converting plasminogen to plasmin which acts on the fibrin of a thrombus but also attacks circulating fibrinogen. These agents are used to treat arterial and venous thrombi. At usual doses, bleeding complications are rare.

If the fibrinolysis must be stopped because of bleeding or the need for an invasive procedure, haemostasis will usually return towards normal within 2 hours of stopping the infusion. More rapid correction can be achieved with infusion of fresh frozen plasma, and cryoprecipitate if the fibrinogen level is extremely low. The use of fibrinolytic inhibitors should be restricted to life-threatening bleeding since excessive clotting may occur. Fibrinolytic therapy is contra-indicated if there is a bleeding history, recent surgery or other risk of bleeding.

Aspirin: Aspirin, even in low dose, produces an irreversible impairment of platelet function by inhibition of cyclo-oxygenase. Because the effect lasts for the lifetime of the platelets (10 days) the impairment of haemostatic function can last several days beyond the cessation of aspirin therapy. This effect can be demonstrated by prolongation of the bleeding time. When an aspirin-induced platelet function defect contributes to bleeding, platelet transfusion is required.

Cardiopulmonary bypass: Bleeding following extra-corporeal circulation may be associated with platelet function defects. Therapy with platelets and fresh frozen plasma is indicated where there is bleeding with laboratory evidence of haemostatic impairment post operatively (following heparin reversal with protamine). The use of DDAVP and Aprotinin to reduce the haemostatic defect of cardiopulmonary bypass is being evaluated.

Congenital haemostatic disorders
Haemophilia. In the United Kingdom patients with Haemophilia A, Haemophilia B and von Willebrand's disease are normally looked after by Regional Haemophilia centres. **The co-operation of the local Regional**

Haemophilia Centre *must* be obtained when a patient with Haemophilia presents to a clinical unit.

Where a haemophiliac presents to a hospital remote from the Regional Haemophilia Centre the following are necessary:

Identification: If the patient is unconscious the information should be present on a bracelet or medallion.

Communication: The Regional Haemophilia Centre should be contacted straight away and will advise on appropriate therapy.

Treatment: Coagulation factor concentrates are needed for Haemophilia A and B. The nearest supply may be the patient's own supply provided for home therapy. Cryoprecipitate is an adequate treatment for Haemophilia A and von Willebrand's disease where factor concentrate is not available. It is not useful in Haemophilia B.

Monitoring: Factor levels may need to be monitored to assess response to treatment and adequacy of dose—this needs a specialist laboratory.

Therapy: Table 7 gives guidance for the levels of coagulation factor activity which may be needed and the doses required to achieve these levels. As a general guide:

  1 iu of factor VIII infused per kg body weight gives an immediate 2% rise in plasma factor VIII level.

  1 iu of Factor IX infused per kg body weight gives an immediate 1% rise in Factor IX level.

Bleeding episodes may be **minor** (haemarthrosis with less than 30% loss of range of motion), **moderate** (severe muscle and joint bleeds, bleeding into gastro-intestinal tract, neck or tongue, and trauma to the head without any evidence of intracranial bleeding); **major** (bleeding that is threatening to life or limb).

Table 7 Treatment of a Bleed in a Haemophilia Patient: Initial Dose of Factor VIII or Factor IX

Severity of bleeding	Recommended trough level of factor (%)	Dose of factor VIII* (iu/kg)	Dose of factor IX† (Iu/kg)
Mild‡ Early joint or muscle bleeding Epistaxis Dental bleeding Persistent hematuria	30	15	30
Moderate‡ Major joint bleeding Muscle bleeding Neck, tongue, pharynx bleeding Gastrointestinal bleeding Suspected abdominal bleeding Head trauma without neurologic deficit	50	25	50
Major§ Intracrancial bleeding Surgery Compartment syndrome Major trauma	75-100	40-50	75-100

* Subsequent doses of Factor VIII are given every 8-12 hrs.
† Subsequent doses of Factor IX are given every 18-24 hrs.
‡ Duration of therapy is determined by time to adequate resolution.
§ Duration of therapy is for minimum of one week but often several weeks.

Von Willebrand's Disease

It is now recommended in the UK that bleeding in patients with Von Willebrand's disease is managed with Factor VIII concentrate. An alternative is infusion of cryoprecipitate: 10-20 bags of cryoprecipitate in an adult, repeated every 8-12 hours as required. Assessment of response and therapeutic requirements are not as straightforward as with Haemophilia A and B. Bleeding time, Factor VIII: C and von Willebrand Factor antigen levels are monitored.

As a general guide, required factor levels are 30% (30 iu/dl) for minor bleeds (function usually restored within 24 hours); 50% for moderate bleeds and 75-100% for major bleeds. **(These figures refer to the trough level—ie the lowest factor level reached before the next infusion must be given.)** To attain the required level enough factor is infused to raise the level immediately to **twice** the target level. Half this dose is then repeated at the half-life time of the factor, that is 8-12 hours for Factor VIII and around 24 hours for Factor IX.

The factor content of Factor VIII and Factor IX concentrates is marked on the vials.

The Factor VIII content of cryoprecipitate is approximately 80 units per bag.

It is emphasised that every effort must be made to obtain immediate specialist assistance in the management of these patients.

Transfusion for patients with bone marrow failure

Treatment of leukaemia and other malignant conditions may lead to periods of profound suppression of the bone marrow during which there is a fall in production of platelets, red cells and white cells.

Because episodes of marrow failure may be repeated or prolonged there are special problems in providing transfusion support.

Thrombocytopenia and platelet replacement: Bleeding in the presence of a platelet count below $50 \times 10^9/l$ will require platelet replacement. High doses (6 units twice daily or more) may be needed particularly if there is concurrent sepsis or DIC. To prevent bleeding, platelets are often given prophylactically to patients with marrow failure whose platelet counts fall below a predetermined level. This level may be set at $20 \times 10^9/l$ although some authorities advise a lower threshold $(10 \times 10^9/l)$ for prophylactic use of platelets when the patient is not febrile.

Granulocyte replacement: (The indications are given in *Section 2*). The use of granulocyte concentrates has declined sharply in recent years as the benefits are limited when appropriate antibiotic therapy is given.

Irradiation of blood components: All cellular blood components contain leucocytes and could potentially cause Graft **versus** Host disease in a recipient with reduced immune defences. Irradiation (1500-2500 cGy) removes the lymphocyte's ability to respond to the recipient's antigens. Patients who have received bone marrow transplantation should receive irradiated cellular blood components. Irradiation should if possible be performed not more than a few hours before infusion since red cell potassium loss increases after irradiation.

CMV testing of blood components: A high proportion of blood donors have serological evidence of past CMV infection (from 50% in some Western countries to 80% in other parts of the world). Some of these donors can transmit CMV to CMV sero-negative patients who are immunosuppressed. In many centres, bone marrow transplant recipients who are themselves CMV sero-negative and who have received a graft from a CMV sero-negative donor are routinely given CMV sero-negative components. The use of leucocyte depleted platelet and red cell preparations may also reduce CMV transmission. Some additional protection against CMV pneumonitis may be obtained by prophylactic administration of CMV immunoglobulin.

Alloimmunisation problems in multi transfused patients: Patients receiving repeated blood component infusions are likely to develop allo-antibodies to blood cells, platelets or plasma proteins. This can happen even in severely immunosuppressed patients.

Platelets: Antibodies to HLA or platelet specific antigens are associated with inadequate responses ('refractoriness') or reactions to platelet infusions. Refractoriness to platelets may develop in up to 50% of leukaemic patients. The incidence of this complication may be reduced by use of leucocyte poor blood components to minimise HLA allo-immunisation. Haemostasis may be achieved in refractory patients by the use of large doses of random donor platelets or single donor (apheresis) platelets from an HLA compatible donor.

A platelet crossmatch (donor platelets with recipient's serum) may give useful evidence about the cause of refractoriness in an individual patient (eg immune or non-immune) but may not be routinely available.

Red cells: Antibodies are detected by routine antibody screening and compatible red cells must be supplied.

White cells: Antibodies to white cells may also lead to pyrexial transfusion reactions caused by the leucocytes present in standard preparations of red cells or platelets. Such patients should nevertheless be checked for red cell antibodies. The majority of patients who experience a pyrexial transfusion reaction will not have a repeat reaction to further component infusions. Patients who do experience a second reaction should receive leucocyte depleted red cell products for all future transfusions (*Page 10*).

Transfusion and transplantation

Transfusion of whole blood or blood components may influence the recipient's immune system and affect the outcome of a transplant. These possible benefits and risks should influence transfusion decisions for patients who may later need transplantation.

Kidney transplantation: Graft survival is improved if the recipient has been transfused with whole blood or red cell concentrate. Most centres therefore have a planned regime of pretransplant transfusion. In some patients transfusion can induce anti-lymphocyte (lymphocytoxic) antibodies which make it difficult to find a compatible kidney donor. Where a live donor is to be used, some centres arrange for the recipient to receive pretransplant transfusions from the kidney donor as this further improves graft survival. The use of cyclosporin has also improved graft survival and this has reduced the extra benefit which can be obtained by pretransplant transfusion.

Bone marrow transplant recipients: It is often immunologically disadvantageous to transfuse the recipient before transplantation because sensitisation to HLA antigens reduces the chance of marrow graft survival, especially in recipients with aplastic anaemia or thalassaemia. Early transplantation in these conditions will reduce the need for blood component support before grafting. Blood components should not be prepared from family members (potential marrow donors). Leucocyte depleted cellular products should be used to minimise exposure to HLA antigens. (Following transplantation, the transfusion problems are those dealt with on *Page 68*).

Immune cytopenias—use of IV IgG

Idiopathic Thrombocytopenic Purpura: Although intravenous immunoglobulin in high doses has a role in the management of some patients, it is not a substitute for the standard treatment including steroids and splenectomy. IV IgG produces increases in platelet count of varying duration in a majority of patients but prolonged responses are more common in acute than in chronic ITP. IV IgG may be used to assist management of acute bleeding when conventional therapy is insufficient. It is useful for covering surgery or delivery in patients with ITP. A daily dose of 0.4-1.0 g/kg is given and total courses of 1 to 2 g/kg over 1-5 days have been used. In some patients, further doses of 0.4 g/kg periodically may maintain an adequate platelet count.

Post transfusion purpura, neonatal allo-immune thrombocytopenia, neonatal thrombocytopenia due to maternal ITP: In all these conditions IV IgG in the dose regimes given above has been shown to produce effective rises in platelet count. In post transfusion purpura, IV IgG is probably the treatment of choice usually in combination with steroids.

Immunoglobulin preparations for prevention and treatment of infection

Both Normal Human Immunoglobulin and a variety of products with higher levels of antibody against specified organisms are used, often together with active immunisation, to protect against infection. A summary of the products and their use is given in *Table 8.*

More detailed guidance is given in the Departments of Health Handbook "Immunisation Against Infectious Disease".

Table 8 The Use of Immunoglobulin Preparations for Prevention of Infection

Infection	Indications	Preparations, vial content	Dose
Hepatitis A	Contacts and travellers	**Normal Human Immunoglobin** (NHIg) 250 mg and 750 mg	Under 10 yrs 250 mg 10 yrs and over 500 mg
Measles	Immuno-compromised, contacts infant contacts with pre-existing severe illness	NHIg 250 and 750 mg (unless **Measles Immunoglobulin** is available)	Under 1 yr 250 mg 1-2 yrs 500 mg 3 yrs and over 750 mg

Immunoglobulin is **not** used with measles vaccine. An interval of at least 3 months must elapse after an injection of immunoglobulin before measles vaccination is attempted.

Rubella	Pregnant contact where termination is not an option	NHIg 750 mg (unless **Rubella Immunoglobin** is available)	750 mg

Normal immunoglobulin after exposure **does not prevent infection and is not generally recommended for protection of pregnant women exposed to rubella.** It may be used when termination of pregnancy would be unacceptable. In this case it should be given without awaiting reports on the woman's serological status. Serological follow-up is essential.

Tetanus	High risk injuries to non-immune subjects	**Tetanus Immunoglobulin** 250 iu	250 or 500 iu

Use together with active (toxoid) immunisation in tetanus prone wounds in the following: (i) unimmunised subjects, (ii) immunisation history unknown, (iii) over 10 years since last tetanus vaccine. Dose 250 iu but use 500 iu if more than 24 hours have elapsed since injury or if there is a risk of heavy contamination.

Tetanus	Clinical tetanus	**Tetanus Immunoglobulin;** 3000 iu vials (if available or 250 iu vials)	30-3000 iu/kg multiple IM sites or IV if suitable product available

Table 8—continued   The Use of Immunoglobulin Preparations for Prevention of Infection

Infection	Indications	Preparations, vial content	Dose
Rabies	Bite or mucous membrane exposure to potentially rabid animals	**Human Rabies Immunoglobulin** (HRIg) 500 iu	20 iu/kg

Rabies immunoglobulin is used with rabies vaccine to provide rapid protection until the vaccine becomes effective. The recommended dose must not be exceeded and should be given at the same time as the vaccine. Half the does should be infiltrated round the wound and the remainder given by deep intramuscular injection at a site separate from that used for rabies vaccine.

Hepatitis B	Needlestab or mucosal exposure. Sexual exposure	**Hepatitis B Immunoglobulin** (HBIg) 500 iu, 1000 iu	1000 iu (or 2 × 500 iu: see note below)

Treat within 48 hours if possible and not more than 10 days after exposure. If 500 iu given initially repeat does at 28 days unless recipient has been shown to be immune or inoculum has come from a low risk (anti-HBe positive) individual or the recipient has received hepatitis B vaccine.

Hepatitis B	Newborn babies of high risk mothers.	**Hepatitis B Immunoglobin** 100 iu	200 iu

As soon as possible and within 48 hours after birth. Combine with simultaneous active immunisation.

Varicella Zoster	Immuno-compromised contacts. Neonatal contacts	**Varicella Zoster Immunoglobulin** (ZIg) 250 mg and 500 mg vials	0-5 yrs 250 mg 6-10 yrs 500 mg 11-14 yrs 750 mg 15+ yrs 1000 mg. (Note these doses recommendations for BPL product: for other product see package insert)

Used in *(1)* chickenpox or zoster contacts if they are immunosuppressed by reason of drugs, radiation, neoplasm or immunodeficiency disease, *(2)* neonates born 6 days or less after the onset of maternal chickenpox or whose mothers develop chickpox (not zoster) after delivery, *(3)* other neonatal contacts of chickenpox or zoster if **either** the baby is very premature (less than 30 weeks gestation or under 1 kg birthweight) or the mother has no prior history of chickenpox, *(4)* if supplies permit it may be given to pregnant contacts to reduce the risk of severe infection.

Table 8—Continued

Other Immunoglobulin Preparations

The following special special preparations are available from Regional Transfusion Centres in Scotland.

Normal Immunoglobulin for intravenous use, Rubella Immunoglobulin, Measles Immunoglobulin, Tetanus Immunoglobulin 3000 Iu pack for Intravenous administration in treatment of established tetanus, Anti CMV Immunoglobulin.

All these products are supplied with package inserts and must be prescribed according to the manufacturer's instructions.

Sources of Supply

England and Wales	**Normal Immunoglobulin: CDSC, Central Public Health Laboratory 01 200 6060 and other Public Health Laboratories. Blood Products Laboratory 01 953 6191.**
	Tetanus Immunoglobulin: Regional Transfusion Centres.
	Hepatitis B Immunoglobulin: Hepatitis Epidemiology Unit, CPHL and other Public Health Laboratories.
	Rabies Immunoglobulin: Virus Reference Laboratory, CPHL.
	Varicella Zoster Immunoglobulin: CDSC AT CPHL.
Scotland	All immunoglobulin products are supplied through the Regional Transfusion Centres.

Immunoglobulin products are also available from commercial suppliers, usually through hospital pharmacies.

Primary hypogammaglobulinaemia—Immuno-globulin replacement

These patients have an inherited deficiency in antibody production and require life-long replacement therapy to avoid or control infectious complications of immune deficiency. Intramuscular immunoglobulin is often poorly tolerated due to pain at the injection site (especially in children) and it may often be impossible to maintain levels of plasma IgG sufficient to prevent recurrent infection. For most patients the treatment of choice is regular administration of IV IgG.

The dosage of IV IgG is 200 mg/kg every three weeks but the dose may require to be increased, or infusions given more frequently if recurrent infections persist and if the plasma IgG level cannot be maintained within the normal range. If IM IgG is used, the standard dose is 25-50 mg/kg weekly. The higher dose requires a very painful IM injection (20 ml for a 60 kg adult).

Therapeutic apheresis

Therapeutic apheresis involves removal of blood or a blood component. The simplest procedure is therapeutic venesection, in which whole blood (450 ml units) is periodically withdrawn. This is indicated for some patients with haemochromatosis or polycythaemia vera. More commonly, cells or plasma are selectively removed using a cell separator. Either discontinuous or continuous flow centrifugal cell separators may be used. Membrane separators can be used only for plasmapheresis.

Indications:
Therapeutic plasma exchange combined with other appropriate medical treatment is used in managing hyperviscosity syndromes, rapidly progressive glomerulonephritis, Goodpasture's syndrome, Guillain-Barré syndrome, familial hypercholesterolaemia, and thrombotic thrombocytopenic purpura. Plasmapheresis has also been used in many other conditions such as myasthenia gravis, pemphigus, SLE, other autoimmune disorders and maternal Rh D sensitisation. Its effectiveness has not been convincingly proved in these conditions and in many cases

objective monitoring is difficult. In view of this, the potential hazards of plasmapheresis should be borne in mind when deciding to use this form of therapy. Good venous access is essential. Some machines can operate using a single vein but normally separate cannulae are required for withdrawal and return.

Replacement fluids include 4.5% albumin, sodium chloride 0.9% or a mixture of these. Fresh frozen plasma should not be used routinely due to the risk of virus infection and acute anaphylactic reactions but may occasionally be needed to correct a deficiency of coagulation factors at the end of the procedure. It should also be used for plasma exchange in the treatment of thrombotic thrombocytopenic purpura.

Cytapheresis: Leukapheresis may be used to reduce viscosity symptoms in leukaemic patients who have a very high white count. Plateletpheresis is occasionally used in patients with platelet counts $> 10^{12}$ per litre who have bleeding or thrombotic problems. Erythrocytapheresis (red cell exchange) may be used in the management of severe malaria, sickle-cell crisis or polycythaemia rubra vera.

Complications of therapeutic apheresis include anaphylactic reactions to fresh frozen plasma, volume overload or hypovolaemia, air embolism, haemolysis, extracorporal clotting, citrate toxicity, coagulopathy, and vasovagal attacks.

Table 9 1989 Prices of Blood Components and Plasma Fractions

Blood Components (Based on Health Departments Handling Charges)	£
Whole Blood	26
Red Cell Concentrate—supplemented	14
Red Cell Concentrate	14
Filtered (leucocyte depleted) Red Cells	28
Platelet concentrate (1 donation)	14
Fresh Frozen Plasma (200-250 ml)	12
Cryoprecipitate (1 donation)	10

Plasma Fractions (Based on Commercial Suppliers' Charges)	£
Albumin 5%, 500 ml	
Albumin 20%, 100 ml	} 35-50
Factor VIII 250 iu	35-75
Factor IX 350-600 iu	35-75
Human Immunoglobulin im 750 mg	7
Human Immunoglobulin iv 5g	75-100
Tetanus Immunoglobulin 1 dose	16
Hepatitis Immunoglobulin 1 dose	40
Anti-D Immunoglobulin 500 iu	15-25

Other Fluids for Volume Resuscitation

Crystalloids		£
Sodium Chloride Intravenous Infusion 0.9% BP	500 ml	0.5
Ringer's Solution for Injection BP	500 ml	0.5

Non Plasma Colloids		
Dextran 40 Intravenous Infusion BP	500 ml	2.5-6.5
Dextran 70 Intravenous Infusion BP	500 ml	4.0-5.0
Haemaccel	500 ml	3.8
Hetastarch	500 ml	15-16
Gelofusin	500 ml	2.5-3.0

The figures cannot be taken as a definitive guide to costs.

Note that 5% albumin costs about 100 times more than saline solution.

Table 10 Telephone/FAX Numbers of Regional Transfusion Centres

	Tel. No.		Fax No.	
North (Newcastle upon Tyne)	(091)	2611711	(091)	2324554
Yorkshire (Leeds)	(0532)	645091/2/3	(0532)	603925
Trent (Sheffield)	(0742)	424242	(0742)	435083
East Anglia (Cambridge)	(0223)	245921		
North West Thames (Edgware)	(01)	9525511	(01)	9514447
North East Thames (Brentwood)	(0277)	223545	(0277)	225662
South London (Tooting)	(01)	6728501/7		
Wessex (Southampton)	(0703)	776441		
Oxford	(0865)	65711		
South West (Bristol)	(0272)	507777	(0272)	508978
West Midlands (Birmingham)	(021)	4141155		
Mersey (Liverpool)	(051)	7097272	(051)	7090392
North West (Manchester)	(061)	2737181	(061)	2743941
(Lancaster)	(0524)	63456	(0524)	62602
Wales (Cardiff)	(0222)	890302	(0222)	890825
North-East Scotland (Aberdeen)	(0224)	681818	(0224)	695351
East of Scotland (Dundee)	(0382)	645166	(0382)	642551
South East Scotland (Edinburgh)	(031)	2292585	(031)	2291069
Glasgow & West of Scotland (Carluke)	(0698)	373315/8	(0698)	356770
North of Scotland (Inverness)	(0463)	232695	(0463)	237020
Northern Ireland (Belfast)	(0232)	321414		

80

Figure 1 Processing of blood from donor to patient.

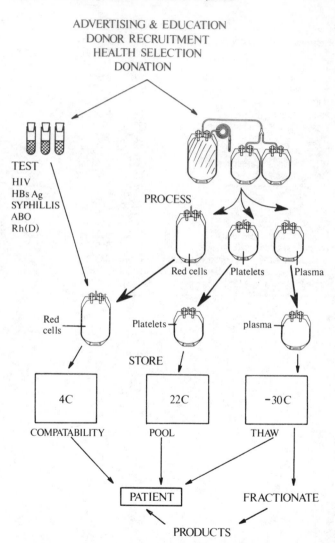

ADVERTISING & EDUCATION
DONOR RECRUITMENT
HEALTH SELECTION
DONATION

TEST

HIV
HBs Ag
SYPHILLIS
ABO
Rh(D)

PROCESS

Red cells   Platelets   Plasma

Red
cells   Platelets   plasma

STORE

| 4 C | 22 C | −30 C |

COMPATABILITY   POOL   THAW

PATIENT   FRACTIONATE

PRODUCTS

Figure 2 Scheme of plasma fractionation.

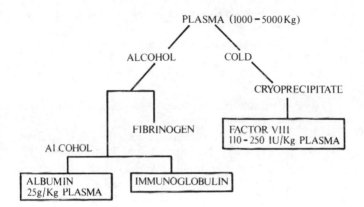

4 DONATIONS PROVIDE 1 bottle of 5% Albumin (20g)
5-6 DONATIONS PROVIDE 1 bottle of Factor VIII (250 iu)

Further reading

Consensus Conference. Fresh-frozen plasma. Indications and risks. JAMA 1985; 253, 551-3.

Consensus Conference. Platelet transfusion therapy. JAMA 1987; 257, 1777-80.

Consensus Conference. Perioperative red cell transfusion. JAMA 1988; 260, 2700-3.

Brozovic, B. and Brozovic, M. Manual of clinical blood transfusion. Edinburgh: Churchill Livingstone, 1986.

Kelton, J.G., Heddle, N.M. and Blajchman, M.A. Blood transfusion. A conceptual approach. New York: Churchill Livingstone, 1984.

Napier, J.A.F. Blood transfusion therapy: a problem orientated approach. Chichester: Wiley, 1987.

Mollison, P.L., Englefriet, C.P. and Contreras, M. Blood transfusion in clinical medicine. 8th ed. Oxford: Blackwell Scientific Publications, 1987.

Bloom, A.L. and Thomas, D.P. eds. Haemostasis and thrombosis. 2nd ed. Edinburgh: Churchill Livingstone, 1987.

Cash, J.D. ed. Progress in transfusion medicine; Edinburgh: Churchill Livingstone, Vol 1: 1986, Vol 2: 1987, Vol 3: 1988.

Guidelines for compatibility testing in hospital blood banks. A joint publication of the British Society for Haematology and the British Blood Transfusion Society. Clin. Lab. Haematol., 9, 333-41, 1987.

Guidelines for transfusion for massive blood loss. A publication of the British Society for Haematology. Clin. Lab. Haematol., 10, 265-73, 1988.

Guidelines on hospital blood bank documentation and procedures. British Society for Haematology, 1984.

Joint Committee on Vaccination and Immunisation. Immunisation against infectious disease. London: Her Majesty's Stationery Office, 1988.

Guidelines for autologous transfusion. A joint publication of the British Society for Haematology and the British Blood Transfusion Society. Clin. Lab. Haematol., 10, 193-201.

Index

88

Printed in the United Kingdom for Her Majesty's Stationery Office.
Dd 0291184, 1/89, C480, 3385/2, 16268.